VACCINOSIS

AND ITS CURE BY THUJA;

VACCINOSIS

AND ITS CURE BY THUJA;

WITH REMARKS ON

HOMŒOPROPHYLAXIS:

BY

J. COMPTON BURNETT, M.D.

GYAN

Published by

Gyan Publishing House
5, Ansari Road
Daryaganj, New Delhi-110002
Phone: 011-47034999, 9811692060
E-mail: books@gyanbooks.com

Distribution Network
gyanbooks.com
India, USA, Canada, UK, Australia, France

ISBN : 978-81-212-6550-8 (PB)
First Published, 1884

2nd Impression 2022

Printed at: Gyan Press, Delhi.

VACCINOSIS AND ITS CURE BY THUJA
Author: J. COMPTON BURNETT

VACCINOSIS

AND ITS CURE BY THUJA;

WITH REMARKS ON

HOMŒOPROPHYLAXIS:

BY

J. COMPTON BURNETT, M.D.

Arbor vitæ: nomen omen.
Similia similibus prævenientur.

1884.

To

THAT EMINENT

CHRISTIAN CITIZEN AND ARDENT CHAMPION

OF LIBERTY,

Rowland Rees, J.P.,

MAYOR OF DOVER,

THE

FOLLOWING PAGES ARE ADMIRINGLY DEDICATED

BY

The Author.

PREFACE.

TRUTH is not Truth save only to the Infinite; to the mind of mortal man Truth is not necessarily Truth, but only that which *appears* to be true. Hence it is that what is a glorious truth to one man is inglorious nonsense to another, and both individuals may be equally honest of purpose and of like earnestness in their search after Truth.

Minds have their affinities no less than matter, and no one ought, after reflection, to be disappointed to find his own most cherished pursuits contemned and ridiculed by men of other minds.

The contents of this little volume appear to the writer to constitute an important elucidation of certain, otherwise obscure, clinical phenomena; for him vaccinosis is a sub-division of the sycosis of Hahnemann; and its recognition of considerable utility in the consulting-room and at the bedside. The idea of using *Thuja Occidentalis* as here recommended is not new, nor is it peculiar to the writer, though it is but very little known in this country, and still less acted upon, and hence it is hoped that the publication of these pages may help to establish vaccinosis as a form of disease, and *Thuja* as one of its chief remedies.

There is an admirable Prize Essay on Thuja, by a learned German physician of eminence, Dr. H. Goullon, of Weimar, entitled "THUJA OCCIDENTALIS. Abendländischer Lebensbaum. Eine monographisch-therapeutische Abhandlung nebst Kritischer Beleuchtung der sogenannten LUES GONORRHOICA (blenorrhoischen Syphilis) oder SYKOSIS HAHNEMANN'S von Dr. Med. H. Goullon." This important essay obtained the prize of the *Homœopatische Centralverein* of Germany, and was published at Leipsic in 1877, by Baumgärtner. It is a complete monograph on the subject of which it treats, and is eminently instructive and suggestive.

In Dr. Goullon's Essay, p. 64, we read "Dr. Kunkel erinnert bei dieser Gelegenheit an die Aehnlichkeit des Krankheitsbildes, wie es die von uns so genannte Vaccinose, d. i. der Complex von Krankhaften Symptomen nach dem Impfen bietet und wie es der eben beschriebene sycotische Tripper darstellt. Auch sei bei beiden das Incubationsstadium verhältnissmässig kurz." And, again, p. 120, "Folgen des Impfens und Revaccinirens."

To those to whom the evidence adduced may be insufficient as proof of the existence of VACCINOSIS, to those, it is submitted, the facts may nevertheless possess some interest merely as a *Contribution to the Clinical History of Thuja Occidentalis.*

And, moreover, if the *Thuja* cured the recorded cases it must be manifest that the efficacy of very minute doses is a factor yet to be reckoned with by practical medicine, both curative *and preventive.*

Of the critics it is merely asked that

they go to their task—*sine ira et studio:* truth is the aim of the writer.

As to the word *vaccinosis* it is only needful to say that, though a hybrid word-form, it is coined on the model of such designations as scrofulosis and tuberculosis, whose sole apology is practical usefulness and the difficulty of putting pure word-forms in their stead.

In regard to the second part of this little treatise on *Homœoprophylaxis* the writer believes it will prove suggestive and instructive, and he is not without some hope that it may lead to a clearer appreciation of how the law of similars might with advantage be extended systematically to the prevention of specific diseases. How far this may be possible experience must shew.

J. COMPTON BURNETT.

5, HOLLES STREET,
CAVENDISH SQUARE, W.,
March, 1884.

On Vaccinosis and its Cure by Thuja Occidentalis, with remarks on Homœoprophylaxis.

FEAR not, critical reader, this is *not* an anti-vaccination treatise, for the writer is himself in the habit of vaccinating his patients, *au besoin*, and he believes that vaccination *does* protect, to a certain large extent, from small-pox, though the protection must necessarily cease as soon as the vaccinated person has slowly returned to his pristine state of pure health.

The writer starts with this declaration just to clear the ground, and to explain that the following pages are neither pro-vaccinational nor anti-vaccinational in the ordinary sense, inasmuch as their scope is essentially one of aetiopathology and cure, and of Homœoprophylaxis.—That is to say: the writer's aim is to shew, 1*st*, that there exists a diseased state of the constitution which is engendered by the vaccinial virus (the so-called lymph), which state he proposes to call VACCINOSIS, or the *Vaccinial State*; and, 2*ndly*, that there exists also in nature a notable remedy for said Vaccinosis, *viz.*: the *Thuja Occidentalis*; and, 3*rdly*, that *Thuja* is a remedy of Vaccinosis by reason of its homœopathicity thereto; *4thly*, that the law of similars also applies to the prevention of disease.

Vaccinosis does not express merely the same thing as *vaccinia*, for the latter means the febrile reaction which occurs in an organism after vaccination, with special reference to the local phenomena at the point where the vaccinial pus, or lymph, is inserted. Sometimes, also, the term vaccinia is applied to a general varioloid eruption following vaccination; but here, vaccinia is commonly held to end.

Now all this is included by me in the term vaccinosis, but still *I do not* mean *merely this, but also that profound and often long-*

lasting morbid constitutional state engendered by the vaccine virus, which virus we usually euphemistically term "lymph." Lymph, of course, it is not, but pus—matter—and why a specific virulent pus should be persistently called "lymph" seems somewhat peculiar, and is eminently unscientific. As I am a lover of purity, and incidentally also of philological purity, I call this "lymph" pus, because it is pus and *not* "lymph." The diseased state, then, engendered by this vaccinial pus, by vaccination, is *vaccinosis*; and in it are *not* included any other diseases whose causes may be accidentally or incidentally contained in the vaccine pus,—such as scrofulosis, syphilis, or tuberculosis.

Wherein does the Protective Power of Vaccination consist?

Given a *perfectly healthy* individual who has never been vaccinated. We say to such a one, you must be vaccinated or you are liable to catch small-pox, which is often about. Let us pause to note clearly that the individual thus warned by us as being liable to catch small-pox *is perfectly healthy*. Now let us vaccinate this perfectly healthy person, and, the vaccination succeeding, we say he is henceforth protected from small-pox. That is to say this thoroughly healthy non-vaccinated person becomes more or less proof against the contagion of small-pox by vaccination, or, at any rate, it is so averred.

It may be safely admitted that no one can be *more* than perfectly healthy, and any modification or altering of perfect health must result in a minus, *i.e.*, *less* than perfect health; and *less* than perfect health must necessarily be disease or ill health of some sort and in some degree.

Hence it follows that the protective power of vaccination is due to a *diseased* state of the body. [See Remarks on Homœoprophylaxis further on.]

Forms of Vaccinosis.

Vaccinosis shews itself as a formidable acute disease that may terminate fatally, or it may manifest itself as a chronic affection. The ordinary forms of vaccinia must be included under acute vaccinosis. The word Vaccinose (Vaccinosis) is used* in the homœopathic literature of Germany, though hardly generally accepted. So far as I know, it has no place in English literature, either homœopathic or general, at all. But the literature of anti-vaccinators teems with examples of "ill-effects of vaccination," "consequences of vaccination," and the like. Most of these would fall under the general term vaccinosis, but only in so far as they are due to "pure" vaccine pus. Here let me remark that it is too often lost sight of that "*pure* vac-

*Thuja Occidentalis, by Goullon (j. cit.).

cine lymph" means vaccine pus (matter) and nothing else, just as we would say *pure* consumption, *pure* syphilis, *pure* poison. The general idea is that *pure* vaccine lymph is as harmless as bread and butter.

Chronic vaccinosis more particularly lies completely beyond the ken of ordinary medicine, and although it will sometimes turn up in literature as "Ill effects of vaccination," it is, nevertheless, but an unrecognised waif, much to the disadvantage of suffering mankind and of medical science. It has not yet been sufficiently studied to be readily* defined; except causally,

* See, however, the writings of Rummel, Bœnninghausen, von Grauvogl, Kunkel, and H. Goullon.

indeed, its very existence is not generally admitted. But a study of the following cases will afford ample evidence that its symptoms are *very like* the pathogenetic symptoms of *Thuja Occidentalis.*

A few preliminary remarks on vaccinosis may here follow before we go to my clinical evidence.

For convenience' sake let us call the vaccinated person a *vaccinate.*

Latent Vaccinosis.

The vaccinate is one who is suffering from vaccinosis ; he may not be ill in the ordinary sense, but he must be in a subdued morbid state, he has been blighted, or he is no vaccinate ; it is his diseased condition that protects him from small-pox.

Some may, perhaps, say that vaccinosis is the same as vaccinia; this is, however, not so; vaccinosis is vaccinia and something more, for if a person is vaccinated unsuccessfully he has *not* had vaccinia, whereas some of the worst cases of (my) vaccinosis which I have met with were just those in whom the vaccination did not "take," as the saying goes. Hence I must call attention to what I believe is a fact, *viz.*: that it often *does* take deep hold of the constitution without calling forth any local phenomena, and, not only so, but such cases may be even very severe in their *internal* developments manifested by the supervention of various morbid symptoms after vaccination. Let us dwell a little on this novel assertion, I was going to say *fact*, yet probably very few will admit that it is a fact at all, but only a fad of mine, since everybody holds that if the vaccination does not "take" the individual has remained uninfluenced by the process of putting vaccine under the cuticle. In other words, when a person is vaccinated and does not take; is, in fact, unsuccessfully vaccinated, it is held that said person is proof against vaccination, and we certify accordingly. Every one believes that the unsuccessfully vaccinated individual has not in any way been affected or altered by the vaccination.

CLOSE AND MINUTE OBSERVA-

TION, HOWEVER, TEACHES ME THAT SUCH IS BY NO MEANS NECESSARILY THE CASE, FOR NOT A FEW PERSONS DATE THEIR ILL HEALTH FROM A SO-CALLED UNSUCCESFUL VACCINATION. My own conception of the thing is just this:—The vaccinated person is poisoned by the vaccine virus; what is called the "taking" is, in point of fact, the constitutional re-action whereby the organism frees itself more or less from the inserted virus. If the person do not "take," AND THE VIRUS HAS BEEN ABSORBED, the "taking" becomes a chronic process—paresis, neuralgiæ, cephalalgiæ, pimples, acne, &c. The less a person "takes," therefore, (in such a case) the MORE is he likely to suffer from chronic vaccinosis, *i.e.*, from the genuine vaccination disease in its chronic form, very frequently a neuralgia or paresis.

Most practitioners will agree that neuralgia is more prevalent now than ever before within the present age, and experience has forced me to ascribe many such cases to vaccinosis.

If my colleagues object to my aetio-pathology of such neuralgiæ, perhaps they will favour us with a more satisfactory one. The word "neuralgia" covers such a multitude of sins in the world of nosology and pathology that my hypothesis is as exact science compared therewith!

But what evidence have I to offer that shall go to shew whether there is such a disease as vaccinosis? or, that being conceded, whether *Thuja* can cure it?

I will first repeat that I do ***not*** claim to be the originator of this clinical application of *Thuja;* Bœnninghausen was, I believe, the first to point out the homœopathicity of *Thuja Occidentalis* to small-pox itself, and thence its use was extended by Kunkel and Goullon to the curation of the ill-effects of vaccination, or vaccinosis as I propose to call it. My attention was first arrested by hearing of Dr. David Wilson's use of Thuja, and then a perusal of Dr. Kunkel's pamphlet and Dr. Goullon's monograph on Thuja shewed me the great importance of *Thuja* as a dynamic antidote to the effects of vaccination.

Let us now pass on to the consideration of some cases of what I call vaccinosis, and of the behaviour of *Thuja* therein.

A Severe Case—A Dying Baby.

Very early in the year 1881, I was called to see a baby in Harley street, about ten weeks old: its mother thought it was dying. She had previously lost babies by death, and knew what a dying baby looked like. The wee patient had begun its life's journey on the bottle; but, being overtaken by the measles, it nearly died, when a wet nurse was obtained and the baby rallied and began to thrive. But a new wet nurse had to be obtained, as the first went dry from over-feeding. The new wet nurse was healthy and strong, but, having gone into the Marylebone workhouse with her own very fine boy, she was re-vaccinated the day before she was removed therefrom to take charge of the patient in question. The baby throve for two or three days, and the mother was just congratulating herself on her success, when one afternoon it went very ill, and getting much worse towards the evening, the mother sent this message to me—"I think baby is dying." I visited the babe in the warm and airy nursery and investigated everything. There was nothing to account for the sudden change. Baby was ghastly white, and in collapse. On questioning the wet nurse as to her own health and state, she remarked that she was quite well (and she looked it, and had a notably good appetite), but she said her re-vaccinated arm "was a little painful." The vesicular stage of the local vaccinial eruption was just at the point of turning to the pustular.

I thought the matter over a little and came to the conclusion that the poor wee thing was, in point of fact, sucking the vaccinial poison from its nurse through the milk. Therefore I gave *Thuja* 6, in pilules, both to babe and nurse, but whether every half-hour or every hour I do not now remember. Calling later in the evening I noticed baby was asleep and looking a little less ghastly. Next morning it was indeed still pale, but practically well; *and the vaccinial vesicles on the nurse's arm had withered*, and they forthwith dried up completely, in lieu of becoming pustular. That baby never looked back, and is now a bonny child.

It is not possible to prove, of course, that this apparently dying baby was suffering from vaccinosis. It lay apparently dying: I feared it would die. But *some* points in connection with this case are incontrovertible. For instance, it is a *fact* that the nurse had been re-vaccinated; it is equally a *fact* that she was suckling the baby; the baby was desperately ill of something; it got *Thuja* and began to mend forthwith. Moreover, and this point is significant, the vaccinial vesicles in the nurse's arm *withered* instead of going on to their usual development. Hence some disturbing influence must have intervened in her organism, and the only thing I know of was the *Thuja.* If the *Thuja* had no effect upon the suckling woman, what made the vaccinial vesicles wither?

Let us suppose that they withered because the milk drained off all the virus. But the baby sucked the milk, and was *very* ill; and the withering of the vaccination vesicles was *synchronous* with the prompt and evident *amelioration* in the child.

But that is only one case, and proves nothing: there are strange coincidences in organismic life as we all know.

Now let me narrate to you another case of acute vaccinosis, but before doing so it might not be amiss to interpolate an observation by Dr. J. T. Harris, of Boston, and published in the New England Medical Gazette, for June, 1883. I quote it entire, because it strengthens my position somewhat; it runs thus:—

A CASE OF TRUE VACCINIA IN A CHILD FOLLOWING THE VACCINATION OF HER MOTHER.

On the 13*th* of February, 1882, I called at the house of Mr. G——, intending to vaccinate his two children, one about three years old, the other a seven months' babe at the breast, whose head, face, arms, and legs were covered with eczema, *crusta lactea*, from which it was suffering severely. Fearing an aggravation of the humour from complication with the vaccination, I declined to operate, giving as my reason that I thought the child was suffering already; that she would be more feverish, irritable, and would require greater care if vaccinated than at present. Although the three-years-old child was troubled with the same form of humour, I vaccinated her, and also the mother. Both vaccinations took, and ran the usual course without much constitutional disturbance. The fifth day after the operation was Mrs. G——'s sickest day. She then had headache, backache, fever, and chill. The vaccination developed normally, but more rapidly than usual.

On the first day of March the baby was more restless and feverish, requiring constant care. On the second day the mother noticed a number of little red pimples upon the child. These increased rapidly upon the face, arms, and legs. I was called to see the little patient on Saturday, the *4th* of March. The little pimples at this time were very numerous, had increased in size; the areola quite red; some swelling; baby feverish; temperature 102. To the question, "What is it, doctor?" I frankly answered, "I do not know, it is not small-pox nor chicken pox. I shall have to wait until it is more fully developed."

On Sunday morning, the fifth day of the fever, the vesicles were forming and more or less filled with lymph, and in the afternoon some were umbilicated. Fresh eruptions were also developing, and upon the face, arms, and legs—those portions of the surface most severely marked with the eczema—the new eruption had become confluent, the whole character of the eruption resembling that of small-pox. There were without doubt between four and five hundred well-defined circular vesicles upon the child during the course of the disease. I invited Dr. Miles to see the case on Sunday afternoon. After a careful examination we concluded that it was a case of vaccinia, communicated to the child through the mother's milk. That there should be no mistake, however, I called upon Dr. McCullom, the city physician, reported the case, and invited him to see the patient with me, which he did on Monday morning. Dr. Martin, of Roxbury, and Dr. Cutler, of Chelsea, also saw the case, and were much interested in it.

On Monday, Tuesday, and Wednesday, the sixth, seventh, and eighth days, there was much swelling of the face, arms, and legs, where it had taken on the confluent form. The little patient was quite feverish and restless. On the seventh, eighth, and ninth days was quite hoarse, and had some difficulty in swallowing. All the symptoms gradually diminished after the ninth day, and many of the scabs were rubbed off. On the seventeenth day very few adherent scabs remained. *Acon.* and *Tart. emetic* were the remedies used.

At the present time, May 14*th*, the

child shows pits, not deep however. The parts where the eruption was confluent are still quite red. The eczema, however, seems to have left for good, and I am in hopes of seeing a good clear skin before many weeks. Although the diagnosis the first few days was obscure, all doubt was removed, and it was pronounced a case of vaccinia communicated from the mother. You will note that on the fifth day after the re-vaccination of the mother the paroxysm of fever occurred, and ten days after the baby was feverish, and the eruption made its appearance one day later. We can therefore call it fourteen days from the time the babe first took the milk impregnated with vaccinia from its mother. If the system can thus be so thoroughly impregnated with vaccinia, may we not also fear various and worse evils from the milk of unhealthy and unclean nurses?

My remark to this instructive experience of Dr. Harris is, that

Thuja Occidentalis was more Homœopathic to the case than *Acon.* and *Ant. tart.* It shows that vaccinia may most probably be sucked by the babe in the milk, though this is not conclusively shewn, inasmuch as it may have been a case of small-pox in the suckling.

The same transmissibility of disease through the milk has been observed more than once. For instance—On Christmas-day last, 1883, M. Layet and a number of medical men, veterinary surgeons, and others, examined and reported on an alleged case of spontaneous cow-pox occurring in a milch cow at Cérons near Bordeaux. The animal presented on the four teats and the neighbouring parts of the udder a considerable number of small pustules, most of them already dried and covered with black crusts, but some containing a more or less milky fluid. The eruption was confluent, and there were no umbilicated pimples. It had made its first appearance on December *22nd*. On December *26th*, six or seven tubes were filled with the fluid from such pustules as had not already burst. The reporters state that an infant fed with the milk from this cow had at the same time presented very similar symptoms.

I now revert to my narrative.

Observation ii.

Acute Vaccinosis.

Aug. *21st*, 1881.—On this day

there was brought to me a little boy, of five months of age, on the bottle, and I was informed that he had been ailing a week, beginning with violent vomiting, loss of appetite, and greenish slimy diarrhœa. The child looked very ill, pale; upper eye-lids drooping; tongue very thickly coated, moist; temperature high; throat severely ulcerated; deglutition painful; on the anterior aspect of the uvula one saw an open ulcer of about the size of a large split pea. The greatest distress lay in the throat; the mother brought him on this account; it pained his throat; which was visibly and demonstrably severely ulcerated: so I gave him *Kali Chloratum* 6, trituration, a dose every hour, and ordered him to be kept in a room with a good fire, and the windows open.

Aug. *22nd.*—I called and found him no worse; more could not be said. He had had a very restless night. He was profoundly weak, hence I gave *Kali Phos.* 6 in alternation with the other medicine.

23rd.—Not quite so weak, but the green slimy diarrhœa continues. To have *Merc. iod.*

24th.—The tongue had begun to clear a little on the left side, but otherwise there was no material change except that he could swallow a little better. Baby was very weak; his mother looked up at me, and the anxious father kept his eyes fixed on my visage, as I sat and studied the little mannikin: he looked very pale and very ill and weak; could not be got to notice anything, but perpetually whined in a piteous little way. I do not know when I ever felt the weight of responsibility greater. Previously I had carefully enquired about the drains, and had ordered the milkman to be changed, and was careful to seek for the real origin of the child's illness, but I could not trace it to anything. The dwelling was healthy, the bottle clean, and there seemed nothing to account for the illness. Suddenly it occurred to me to ask when the child had been vaccinated. The answer was, on the *12th* July. I learned also that the child had a very bad arm, and that the present illness commenced on the day on which the last vaccinial scab fell off the arm. This shed a light upon the case and allowed its true aetio-pathology to be understood. The disease evidently was an en-exanthem, an eruption on the lining membrane of the throat and gut, due to the vaccination; and the vomiting, diarrhœa, and sore throat started just as these inside pustules broke and discharged their contents, and the feverishness was synchronous therewith. The child's organism had essayed to free itself from the vaccinial poison by an eruption on the internal mucous membrane. Had the child been stronger the eruption would probably have been on the skin in the form of an exanthem simply. I prescribed *Thuja Occi-*

dentalis 30, one-drop powders, one every two hours, and no other medicine.

25th.—Much better, began to mend (in the mother's opinion—and what more competent?) "very soon after the first powder." Has slept better. To continue the *Thuja* powders.

28th.—I called to say good-bye, and found the little one still rather weak, but well and cheerful, and at play on his mother's lap.

Here, *Thuja* 30 brought health to the child and joy to the home.

Of course this case is not conclusive either; for the effects of the vaccination—my vaccinosis—may have been working off, and the fact of the sudden amelioration immediately after the exhibition of the *Thuja* may have been a mere coincidence. Pretty well all *acute* cases are open to this objection, and hence I will relate no more cases of acute vaccinosis: they prove nothing, it can merely be a question of probabilities. *I* am satisfied that these two cases were genuine examples of acute vaccinosis, and that the *Thuja* cured them, but others will, perhaps, demand further proof before they believe either in vaccinosis or in *Thuja* as its cure.

So let us pass on to the consideration of some chronic cases of the vaccinial state, or vaccinosis. For the sake of reference let us number the observations. Two I have narrated, and so we come to

Observation iii.

PUSTULAR ERUPTION.

Mr. J——, a hale-looking, middle-aged London merchant, came under my observation on November 3*rd*, 1881. Said he, "I am not a homœopath, but twenty years ago I had eczema, and the allopaths could not touch it, so I went to a homœopathic doctor, and he cured me." And he went on to say that he believed in homœopathy for skin diseases. On the left leg he had a pustular eruption due, he believed, to a bruise. He had also eczema of the ear, and he volunteered the information that ever since his second vaccination he had been subject to eczema. The eczema of twenty years ago was soon after the re-vaccination.

℞ *Thujæ Occidentalis* 30. Four three-drop powders to the two dozen. To take one, dry on the tongue, three times a day.

He came in a week nearly well; the pustules had at once begun to wither.

The *Thuja* was repeated, but in less frequent dose, and the patient subsequently sent word by his brother to say that his skin was well, and he himself too busy to shew himself as he had promised.

This case also proves nothing, because anyone might get a pustular eruption after a bruise, or without a bruise, and be quickly rid of it, without either suffering from vaccinosis, or getting *Thuja*, supposedly, to cure it. The fact is it is exceedingly difficult to absolutely prove anything clinically at all. The patient himself attributed his cure to the powders, knowing of old the very stubborn nature of all his cutaneous eruptions.

Observation iv.

PUSTULAR ERUPTIONS.

Miss ——, *aet.* 18, was re-vaccinated in July, 1881, at her parents' country residence, thirty miles from London, by the local surgeon, with "lymph" direct from the calf. The operation was very successful, and she had a very "fine" arm. But as the "arm" was just at its greatest perfection she got an eruption on her chin covering its whole extent and involving the lower lip. The thing was very unsightly and had a singularly ugly repulsive aspect. The gentleman who had done the re-vaccination was of opinion that Miss ——— had got some of the vaccine virus on to her finger-nails and inoculated herself by scratching. The sequel, however, shewed that the chin manifestation was from within. The surgeon had ordered applications, two of which were vaseline and zinc ointment, but the eruption on the chin was not to be got rid of. The young lady had to wear a dense veil to hide her face when driving out. She was brought to London for my advice, and I gave *Thuja* 30. In a fortnight she was out and about, and only some diffused redness of the skin remained, but no scar or thickened skin. Now, it might be objected to this case that the *Thuja* had nothing to do with the disappearance of the eruption, because it was just the history of the disease: it ran through its natural course and died. I thought that to myself at the time of prescribing it, but against this was the fact that the arm had healed already, and it had depassed the natural course of vaccinia by at least a fortnight when I first prescribed the *Thuja*. But to have a test I gave her brother, who also had a somewhat similar pustular eruption (and who had been re-vaccinated at the same time), but more spare, and instead of being on the chin, it was around the left nostril. I say, to have a test, I gave this brother of Miss ———, *Antimonium tart.*, which is also, as every one knows, apparently homœopathic to such a pustular eruption. This boy's case will be

Observation v.

This is the brother of Miss ———. (*observ. iv.*)

The two eruptions were similar, though the boy's was comparatively trivial, and of the same age, and from the same cause, *i.e.*, from the vaccine virus. The patients went into the country, and in two or three weeks' time the mother wrote that the young lady was quite well, "the medicine soon put her right" was her expression, but the boy had "a bad cold in his head; nose-bleed; left side of nose swelled and red; two little spots of matter, the size of a large pin's head, at the edge of the nostril, and below it, having something the look of ———'s chin; his arm is also not well, and he has had four little pocks about the vaccination marks." I sent *Thuja* 30, and he was reported well in ten days.

If anyone can account for the cure of these two cases independently of the *Thuja*, his ingenuity is greater than mine. That they were causally connected with the re-vaccination admits of no doubt whatever. Nevertheless, it does not do to be quite sure of one's facts; sources of error are often very occult.

Observation vi.

Post-orbital Neuralgia of twenty years' standing.

This case (which came under observation on January 9*th*, 1882,) is one of considerable interest on various accounts. Its subject, a lady of very high rank, over fifty years of age, had been in turns, and for many years, under almost all the leading oculists of London for this neuralgia of the eyes, *i.e.*, terrible pain at the back of the eyes, coming on in paroxysms and confining her to her room for many days together; some attacks would last for six weeks. Some of the neuralgic pain, however, remained at all times. Her eyes had been examined by almost every notable oculist in London, and no one could find anything wrong with them structurally, so it was unanimously agreed and declared to be *neuralgia of the fifth nerve.* Of course no end of tonics, anodynes, and alteratives had been used. The oculists sent her to the physicians and these back again to the oculists. The late Dr. Quin and other leading homœopaths had been tried, but "no one had ever touched it."

Latterly, and for years, she had tried nothing; whenever an attack came on, she would remain in her darkened bedroom, with her head tied up, bewailing her fate.

To me she exclaimed "My existence is one life-long crucifixion!"

I should have stated that the neuralgia was preceded and accompanied by influenza. In the aggregate these attacks of influenza and post-orbital neuralgia confined her to her room nearly half the year. In appearance she was healthy, well-nourished, rather too much *embonpoint*, and fairly vigorous. A friend of hers had been benefited by homœopathy in my hands, and she therefore came to me "in utter despair."

These are the simple facts of the case, though they look very like piling up the agony! Now for the remedy. The resources of allopathy had been exhausted, and, moreover, I have no confidence in them anyway; homœopathy—and good homœopathy too, for the men tried knew their work—had also failed. Do-nothing, now much in vogue, had fared no better. I reasoned thus: This lady tells me she has been vaccinated five or six times, and being thus very much vaccinated, she may be just suffering from chronic vaccinosis, one chief symptom of which is a cephalalgia like hers, so I forthwith prescribed *Thuja* (30). It cured, and the cure has lasted till now. The neuralgia disappeared slowly; in about six weeks (February 14, 1882) I wrote in my case book "The eyes are well!"

As I have not heard from the patient for some time, I am just writing a note to her to know whether the neuralgia has thus far (December 30, 1882) returned. The reply I will add.

Of course, it does *not* follow that because *Thuja* cured this case of neuralgia of some twenty years' standing that *therefore* the lady was suffering from *vaccinosis*; that *Thuja* DID cure it is incontrovertible, and my vaccinosis hypothesis led me to prescribe it. More cannot be maintained. At least the case must stand as a clinical triumph for *Thuja* (30)—this much is absolute.

In reply to my enquiry, I received the following:

"Jan. 1, (1883).

. . . "I have been in very much stronger health ever since I crossed your threshold, and excepting one or two *attempts* at a return from the enemy, I have been quite free from suffering." . .

This lady continues well of her post-orbital neuralgia at the time of going to press. After the disappearance of the neuralgia she had several other remedies from me for dyspeptic symptoms.

I shall probably never have a more severe case of what I conceive to be vaccinosis than the one just narrated, or one that had lasted longer. Twenty years may be considered enough to declare it *en permanence*, and its gradual cessation within six weeks from the time of commencing with the *Thuja* stamps it as an undoubted drug-cure.

However, the following is not uninteresting.

Observation vii.

Chronic Headache of nine years' duration.

Miss G——, *aet.* 19, came under my care on March 12, 1881, complaining of bad attacks of headache for the past nine years. She said it was as if the back of her head were in a vice, and then it would be frontal, and throbbing as if her head would burst. She was very pale, and her forehead looked shiny and in places brown.

These "head attacks" occurred once or twice a week.

Tendency to constipation; menses regular; an old sty visible on left eyelid; poor appetite; dislikes flesh-meat ; liver enlarged a little ; had a series of boils in the fall of 1880.

Feet cold ; used to have chilblains. For years cannot ride in an omnibus, or in a cab, because of getting pale and sick ; skin becomes rough in the wind ; lips crack ; gets fainty at times.

To have *Graphites* 30.

April 13*th*. — Appetite and spirits better, but otherwise no change ; questioned as to the duration of the head attacks, she tells me the last but one continued for three weeks—the last, three days. Over the right eye there is a red, tender patch ; *has two or three white-headed pustules* on her face.

Was vaccinated at three months, re-vaccinated at seven

years, and again at fourteen. Had *small-pox about ten years ago.*

Thus here was a case that had had small-pox ten years ago, or thereabouts, for she could not quite fix the date, and had been vaccinated three times besides, once subsequent to the small-pox!

℞ *Tc. Thujæ Occidentalis*, ʒiv. 3*x*.

To take five drops in water twice a day.

May 13*th*.—Much better: has only had one very slight headache lasting an hour or two; the frontal tender patch is no longer tender; no further faintiness at all. Lips crack. The pustules in the face gone and skin quite clear.

To have *Thuja* 12, one drop at bedtime.

June 17*th*.—Was taken ill yesterday fortnight with soreness of stomach; fever; nausea and perspiration. Subsequently spots broke out like pimples,—eight on the face, one each on the thumb and wrist, one on the foot, and two on the back,—they filled with matter, were out five days, became yellow, and then died away. Her mother says the symptoms were just the same as when patient had the small-pox. Her headaches were well just before this bout came on.

July 1*st*.—Continues well.

27*th*.—The headaches have not returned.

Feb. 24*th*, 1882.—The cure holds good, for she has had no headache and is otherwise well. She had subsequently some other remedies for the little tumour on her eyelid and for a small exostosis on lower jaw, but she had received nothing but *Thuja* when the cephalalgia disappeared and it was two or three weeks before the next medicine followed.

Some months after this date this young lady was brought by her mother merely to shew me how well she was, and to take final leave of me; two years later I learned from her mother that she continued well, so the cure is permanent.

An interesting feature in this case is the curious attack which came on at the beginning of June. My reading of it is that it was really a proving of *Thuja*, or a general organismic reaction called forth by it; and this sent me often up to the thirtieth dilution in my subsequent use of *Thuja*, though I have occasionally found the third decimal dilution answer better than the thirtieth.

But this is not the point of my thesis, for this case was evidently cured by the low dilution, and when the low dilutions cure, and cure promptly, even though not very agreeably, but well, it cannot be necessary to go up any higher, especially as one's faith is sufficiently on the stretch without it.

Observation viii.

ENLARGED GLANDS.

APEX-CATARRH.

Master C———, *aet.* 11½, came under my care on August 18*th*, 1881, complaining of a cough, worse at 7-30 p.m.; he also coughed by day and through the night, but it did not wake him. He perspired fearfully, worst on the head, and worse during the night. Over upper half of left lung one heard moist crackling *râles*. The cervical lymphatic glands at the top of the apex of left lung were indurated and distinctly "feel-able." He weighed 5*st.* 4*lbs.* The vaccination scars were on the left arm, and the glands over the apex of right lung were not indurated. Induration of the lymphatics on the left side of the neck (the vaccination being performed on that side), is the rule after vaccination, as anyone may observe for himself if he will take the trouble to examine a *healthy* child just before vaccination and any time thereafter. I say: *any time thereafter*, for the thing generally persists for a very long time unless cured by medical art.

℞ *Thujæ* 30, m. ii. Sac. lac. q.s. Fiat pulv. Tales xxiv. One, three times a day.

Aug. 27*th*.—Is well of cough, but the sweats continue. To take no medicine.

Sep. 6*th*.—The most careful examination of chest reveals no *râle;* there is no cough; the sweats have quite ceased; the said cervical lymphatics can *not* be found. The boy now weighs 5*st*. 8*lbs*., so that he has gained 4*lbs*. in weight since he got the *Thuja*.

Discharged cured.

The boy had been at school, and was sent home to his parents by the school physician on account of his obstinate cough, and because his general symptoms excited alarm. To me it appeared to be the first stage of phthisis. That the boy should increase in weight at home just after returning from school is, of course, not necessarily due to the medicine; home life, too, would improve his nutrition generally, and would perhaps also account for the disappearance of the apex-catarrh, cough, and perspirations. But what is to account for the disappearance of the induration of the cervical glands?

Of course this case offers but little evidence of the existence of vaccinosis or of its cure by *Thuja*; so I will ask the reader to wade through yet a few more observations which I transcribe from my case books. For if there be such a disease as vaccinosis, in other words if vaccination have any ill-effects beyond those commonly epitomized under the name vaccinia, it is clearly important that it should be recognized, and, its existence being demonstrated, it is desirable that we know how to cure it.

Observation ix.

Hairless Patches on Chin.

Mr. ———, a London merchant, came under my care on July *27th*, 1882, to be treated for some roundish hairless patches on either side of his chin, which began four months ago. The larger patch on the right side was about the size of a florin. Had also an old hordeolum on his right lower eye-lid.

Has been twice vaccinated, the second time, twelve years ago, did *not* "take."

℞ *Thujæ Occidentalis* 30 (4 in 24). To take one, dry on the tongue, at bedtime.

Sept. *7th.*—The bald patches are smaller, the one on the left side nearly gone. Has, apparently, a very bad coryza—?—organismic reaction?

Rep.

Oct. *17th.*—The bald patches are gone; the old hordeolum also gone. The closely-shaven beard is now uniform, the previously-existing white bald patches being completely covered with hair.

I give this as an interesting

cure by *Thuja*, but I am not very sure that the disease was really due to vaccinosis because of other points in his clinical history. Still it might have been so, as the hair is very powerfully influenced by the vaccine poisoning. Thus Kunkel observed both a very weak growth of hair, and an excessive growth, especially in wrong places, as effects, he believed, of vaccination. Therefore let it stand as a doubtful case of vaccinosis for what it may be worth,—but there can hardly be any reasonable doubt as to the cure of the case by *Thuja*.

Here it might not be amiss to observe casually that the presence of sties on the eyelids is often, in my opinion, a symptom of vaccinosis. This case is not without practical importance, inasmuch as hodiernal medicine hands over a sty to the chirurgeon's art; and all the time, poor old dame, weens herself so very much superior to scientific therapeutics usually called homœopathy. The conceit of the orthodoxly ignorant is truly sickening.

Observation x.

Habitual Influenzas. General Ill-health and Headache.

Mr. ———, a city gentleman, came under my observation on December 28*th*, 1882, complaining that he was suffering from a series of neglected colds. He is costive; gets boils and pimples; has a number of warts, both flat and pedunculated; never had gonorrhœa; has severe frontal headache these three months; much pain across chest; and feels so out of health that he can no longer attend to his work, which is only light office work. He especially asks for a preventive for his frequent influenza colds. Flesh is flabby and skin spotted with pimples.

The *habitual influenza*, the *chronic frontal headache*, the *pimply skin*, the *feeling of general malaise* point, according to my experience, to vaccinosis. But had patient been vaccinated? Yes. Four times, and did *not* "take" the last *three* times. I do not expect many to agree with my theory that, when an individual is unsuccessfully vaccinated, he may have been seriously affected in his health by the re-actionless vaccination, perhaps more so than as if it had "taken." But it is a *settled* point with me, and in these cases I find *Thuja* as promptly efficacious as in the ordinary forms of vaccinosis.

℞ *Thujæ Occidentalis* 30 (4 in 24). One at bedtime and on rising.

January 10*th*, 1883.—Wonderful improvement already in the first week; the headaches gone (had had them three months), pain in chest gone; and the bowels are less costive. What a change in twelve days!

℞ *Thujæ Occidentalis* 100, as before.

February 8*th*.—Well; he complains of nothing, and merely calls to thank me.

This case made a considerable sensation in the gentleman's large office-circle, partly because the change in his condition was so sudden and complete, and partly because he came to homœopathy demonstratively unwillingly, and in consequence of the earnest solicitations of his *chef de bureau.*

Observation xi.

ACNE OF FACE AND NOSE, AND NASAL DERMATITIS.

A young lady, about twenty years of age, was brought by her mother to me on October 28*th*, 1882. Patient had a very red pimply nose, not like the red nose of the elderly bibber, or like that due to dyspepsia or to tight-lacing, but a pimply, scaly nasal dermatitis, which extended from the cutaneous covering of the nose to that of the cheeks, but appearing here more as facial acne. The nasal dermatitis was, roughly, in the form of a saddle. Of course this state of things in an otherwise pretty girl of twenty was painfully and humiliatingly unpleasant to her and to her friends, in fact it was likely to mar her future prospects very materially, more especially as it had already existed for six years and was making no signs of departing. She also complained of obstinate constipation. The pimples of the nose and face used to get little white mattery heads. In trying to trace the skin-affection back to its real origin I ascertained that the patient was re-vaccinated six years ago, but she could not remember whether the nose was previously affected or not. This re-vaccination was unsuccessful, *i.e.*, it did *not* "take."

℞ *Thujæ Occidentalis* 30.

November 30*th*.—Pimples of face decidedly better. Nose less red. Constipation no better.

℞ *Thujæ Occidentalis* 100.

January 3*rd*, 1883.—The face is free! Her mother gratefully exclaims, "She is wonderfully better." I ask the young lady which powders did her *most good*; she says, "The *last*." The skin of the nose is normal, but the constipation is no better, and for this she remains under treatment.

That *Thuja* cured this case is incontrovertible, but that it was a case of vaccinosis is not quite so certain, though it is far from improbable. The re-vaccination and inflammation of the skin of the nose were referred both to six years ago when she was in Switzerland at school; but patient could not remember which was the first, the bad nose or the vaccination.

Observation xii.

NEURALGIA OF RIGHT EYE.

Mr. ———, a gentleman of position and means, about fifty years of age, came to consult me on 28*th* June, 1882, for a neuralgia of the right eye. He had come in consequence of the cure of the case recorded here as Observation *vi*.

He complained of almost constant pain in right eye ever since Christmas, 1881, *i.e.*, just about six months. Had had neuralgia in head and shoulders in 1866, and so much morphia had been injected in his shoulders by a doctor in Scotland that it almost killed him: for seven or eight hours it was doubtful if he would recover.

Has a brown, eczematous, itchy (at night,) eruption on both shins and between the toes. The neuralgia of right eye, and for which he comes to me, is bad both by day and night, but rather worse at night. Mr. (now Sir William) Bowman had examined the eye and declared it to be neuralgia, the eye being normal.

Mr. White Cooper had done the same.

On my enquiring when he was last vaccinated, he seemed completely frightened, and stammered out rapidly, "I should not like to be vaccinated again."

"Why?"

"I was very seedy the last time I was vaccinated, in fact I felt awfully ill for about a month," and he again hurriedly protested that he would not like to be vaccinated again. The vaccination that had made him so ill was either in 1852 or 1853.

This seemed to me to be a case of vaccinial neuralgia, and therefore I ordered *Thuja* 30, in infrequent dose. This was on the 28*th* of June, 1882.

July 8*th*.—But very little pain after the first powder. To have the same medicine again.

The cure proved permanent, and is interesting as proof of the rapidity with which the *most like* remedy can cure a neuralgia. And, considering how "awfully ill" he had been after his last vaccination, I think it rather probable that this case is an example of vaccinosis.

What do you think ?

Having narrated some rather striking cases of what I conceive to be the neuralgia of vaccinosis, let me pass on to a case shewing evident tissue change or organic disease. It will be

Observation xiii.

Being a case of

DISEASED FINGER-NAILS.

On December *22nd*, 1882, a young lady of 26 came under my care for an ugly state of the nails of her fingers. Naturally a lady of her age would not be indifferent to the state of her nails. These nails are indented rather deeply, and in addition to these indentations there are black patches on the under surfaces of the nails, reaching into the quick. Very slight leucorrhœa occasionally. She had chicken-pox as a child of eleven. On her shoulders there is an eruption of roundish patches forming mattery heads. Has been vaccinated three different times; the last time two years ago, and the nails have become diseased *since* this last vaccination. The black patches have existed these eighteen months.

Looking upon this diseased condition of the nails as evidence of chronic vaccinosis I ordered her *Thuja* 30 (one in 6).

March 19*th*, 1883.—Has continued the *Thuja* 30 for just about three months, with the result that within a fortnight from commencing with it the black patches under the nails began to disappear, and there is now no trace of them. The indentations are notably better. The eruption on the back has not been modified, and for this she remains under treatment; but I thought this much of a case of nail disease would be of some interest, and the more so as it is not easy to demonstrate drug-action on nail growth at all.

We will now go back to the head and the central nervous system.

Observation xiv.

Case of Ptosis.

A young lady of about 25 years of age came to me in May, 1881, telling me that she had had some tooth-stumps extracted in November, 1880, whereafter there was hæmorrhage for eight or nine hours. Two very able men in the homœopathic ranks had treated her for some time with much benefit, but she still remained ill. *Conium* had been of greatest use. She still complained of ptosis of left side;

sleeplessness; reeling to the right when walking out of doors, tendency to fall to the right. I gave her *Equisetum hyemale* (3^x) because her tongue was cracked. (Clinicians may note this *valuable* little wrinkle, *i.e.*, *cracked tongue=Equisetum*, of which I first saw an account in the *Therapeutic Gazette.*) It was continued for months with very great benefit, and was followed by *Bellis per.*, and then by *Juglans regia*, &c. Then came *Avena sativa* θ, *Cadmium* 6 and 12, and *Psoricum* 30, and finally *Titanium* 30.

These more or less well-chosen remedies wrought a great change in the patient, but on the *29th* July, 1882, she still complained that the left eye was wrong. It made her feel sea-sick when she read; pains in left eye worse in the early morn; some ptosis of left upper lid; eye-ball stiff, and an aching across it and right across the forehead, and she was giddy in walking about.

The case having thus come to a standstill, I cast about for some aetiologico-therapeutic *appui*, and in so doing learned that she had been vaccinated four times in all; the last time, three years ago, took but faintly.

Thuja 30 soon cured the ptosis and the other described symptoms.

Of course I cannot prove that we had here to do with a case of vaccinosis, but such it appeared to me. Well-chosen remedies had greatly benefited the patient, but there seemed to be a bar to the complete cure, and *Thuja* effectually removed this bar.

In chronic disease, when the right remedies seem barred in their action, Hahnemann, on the off-chance that it might be due to psora, recommended his disciples to interpose sulphur as the great, most likely, anti-psoric. Most of us have found this a very valuable clinical suggestion, Similarly, I have found that vaccinosis frequently bars the way, and then *Thuja* comes in with simply the beautiful effect of a genuine *simillimum*.

I shall narrate several more such cases before I take my leave, so that others may be in possession of evidence sufficient to form a judgment on the questions of whether there exists such a morbid state as vaccinosis? and whether *Thuja* can cure the same?

Observation xv.

Paresis.

Mr. ———, a private gentleman, married, and one who had always led a healthful life, but too great a traveller, came under my observation early in the year 1882, in a very weak condition. He had had slight hemiplegia of the right side, and still shewed some symptoms of paralysis, *e.g.*, weakness of right arm, occasional dragging of the legs, loss of memory, impaired vision, and loss of power generally. His effective virility was extinct, and had been so for two or three years, and naturally this did not tend to raise his spirits. I treated him for a few months with but slight benefit, when one day he complained of a frontal headache that at once reminded me of the Thuja headache. I gave him *Thuja occidentalis* 30 (4 in 24) and within a few days he remarked a very notable improvement, feeling better than he had for three years. Getting this report at his next visit, I fell to questioning him about vaccination, which I had previously not done: and what was the answer?

Feb. 24*th*, 1883.—"How many times have you been vaccinated?"

"I have been vaccinated six or seven times."

"Did it take every time?"

"No, never."

And from close questioning I satisfied myself that this gentleman had been *six* times *un*successfully vaccinated, and this suggested to me that he was really suffering from that vaccinial blight which I have ventured to call vaccinosis.

Patient had received only four doses of the *Thuja* 30 in the early part of January, 1883, just to cure his headache, and which resulted, *inter alia*, in a hypopubic resurrection of great importance; and the headache having simultaneously left him, he then took the constitutional remedy I had prescribed, *viz.*, *Titanium*, and continued it until a few days ago. I had instructed him to take the *Thuja* only for a few days, till his headache disappeared.

Now, thought I, we will saturate him with *Thuja* and extinguish the vaccinosis; so I gave him this prescription:

℞ *Tc. Thujæ Occidentalis* 3, ℥iv. To take four drops in water night and morning, and report in a month.

The result was quite satisfactory, and he became, in his wife's words—"quite a different man;" all paralytic symptoms having disappeared, and the old headache had not returned at the end of 1883, when I last saw him.

Loss of virile power is frequently a result of vaccination, and when the local debility is due to this cause it is really wonderful how the case is altered by a few doses of *Thuja*.

Observation xxi.

Case of Spinal Irritation.

Miss ——, *aet.* 29, came under my care in November, 1882, complaining of owning a spine. She had been under the best physicians and surgeons of London. Had derived a little benefit from many, most, she thought from the movement cure, under Dr. Roth, of Wimpole Street. She also alleged that mesmeric passes had eased her a good deal.

Her symptoms were legion; she was bent forward, could scarcely walk, her spine very tender and painful; twitchings; pain all down the back; and chilliness, worse at night. Her liver was decidedly enlarged and there was pain in the right side. This hepatic disturbance was righted by *Chelidonium majus* 1; five drops, in water, twice a day. Then, on December 19*th*, I gave her *Kedron* 1, which certainly eased the cephalalgia and chilliness a good deal, and it was therefore continued till

February 9*th*, 1883, when I went into her case a little more thoroughly as to its anamnesis. She had been vaccinated four times successfully, once it did *not* take.

℞ *Thujæ Occidentalis* 30.

March 8*th*.—Patient exclaimed .... "that is capital stuff; I am *very* much better; my back is very much better; the coldness is gone; I am so much stronger altogether."

Rep.

March 31*st*.—Back "wonderfully better."

She needed several other remedies, but practically her cure was effected by *Thuja*.

On May 17*th* she had *Thuja* 100 and soon afterwards began to play at lawn-tennis.

On June 12*th* she reported herself thus—"I have not been so well for three or four years; I feel strong, and can do anything."

I do not know whether any one will admit that this was a case of vaccinosis; certain it is that she had been vaccinated five times and was very ill, practically an invalid, till I gave her *Thuja*, and then she mended and is now well and comparatively vigorous.

Observation xvii.

Case of Scrivener's Cramp; Cephalalgia, and Enlarged Spleen.

Miss ———, *aet.* 29, a city clerk, came under my observation on May *7th*, 1883, complaining of much epigastric beating, pain in left side, great chilliness, and writer's cramp of the right side. An examination shewed an enlargement of the spleen, and a swelling of the left ovary of about the size of a hen's egg. Her breath is heavy, and she gets *giddiness*. She has *frontal headache* of a severe kind almost every day for a long time.

℞ *Ceanothi Americani* 1. Five drops, in water, three times a day.

May 30*th*.—Side is much better; the chilliness is better; the feet warmer; the beating less.

Rep. et *Cup. acet*. I.

July 30*th*.—Side nearly well; paining every alternate day or so. Pain in the back no better; giddiness better. Complains especially of the severe frontal headache, and the cramps in the right arm are so bad that she has had to give up office work.

Has been vaccinated three times, but the last time it did *not* take.

℞ *Tc. Thujæ Occidentalis* 30, night and morning.

August 16*th*.—Headache and writer's cramp well. She returns to work.

November 16*th*.—Continues at

office work with comfort; no return of either headache or cramps. Continues under treatment for ovarian tumour, and gets *Silicea* 6.

The hydrogenoid constitution of von Grauvogl was here well pronounced, and what I call vaccinosis was implanted on it. The action of *Thuja* was most marked, prompt, and durable. Questioned on November 16*th* as to which medicine cured the headache and the cramps, she instantly said it was the powders (*i.e.*, the *Thuja*).

Observation xviii.

Arrested Development and Hemiparesis.

Miss ——, *aet.* 16, was brought to me on May 16*th*, 1883. This was her state: roof of mouth very much arched; left side of face drawn to the left so that her mouth is awry. She speaks very badly; cannot articulate properly; and is very deaf. Has always been so. Has a polypus in left nostril; the tonsils are enormously hypertrophied; breathes very loudly. Left mamma smaller than the right; left side of thorax generally smaller than the right. Tongue is cracked; pain in left side for years; frontal headache for a twelvemonth. Menses normal, having begun six months ago. She was vaccinated at the age of three months; it did not take, and so she was done a second time in both arms, when it took fairly well.

Patient is the child of healthy parents, and there did not appear to be anything to account for the extraordinary backwardness. I reasoned that the child had evidently been blighted by the vaccination, *for she did not readily take* (the organism resisted), and then did take (organism overcome).

℞ *Thujæ Occidentalis* 30. Two drops, daily, for four weeks.

Now note the sequel, not forgetting that the child's condition had been, as described, *nearly all her life*.

June 13*th*.—On this day her mother brought her and reported—this is the note in my case book: "on the whole very much better; can certainly articulate better!! and the head and face are not so onesided, and she hears better!!"

Both parents were agreed that

the changes had been wrought since the medicine had been taken. The father is an unusually gifted professional man, and the mother an educated lady.

Rep.

July 11*th*.—Headache well; side pain better; and the whole state is better. Considering the vaccinial blight removed I gave *Ceanothus Americanus* 1, five drops, in water, night and morning, for two months. I gave this because the spleen was enlarged, *and I thought its specific influence on the left side generally* might be beneficial. I was not disappointed, but very much gratified to see that the left side of thorax began to *grow*, and also the left mamma. The little play of the imagination here as to the leftsidedness of the action of *Ceanothus* was fruitful.

September *7th.*—The increased dulness on percussion in the left hypochondrium having disappeared, and the left side having been manifestly bettered, and that considerably, I reverted to the *Thuja*, and this time gave it in the hundredth centesimal dilution.

October *7th.*—Under this date I read in my case book—"Side remains well, but she seems to have suffered a good deal generally while taking the *Thuja* 100. She articulates *decidedly* better, speaks now so that I can understand her, and her hearing is greatly improved." She remains under treatment, and will receive other constitutional remedies, but the influence of the *Thuja* upon her has been most marked and remarkable. I have myself no doubt that the child's condition of hemiparesis arose from the vaccinial blight, *i.e.*, from *vaccinosis*, she being originally delicate, particularly her nervous system.

Observation xix.

NEURALGIA OF EYES OF NINE YEARS' STANDING.

Miss ———, *aet.* 20, came to me on January 18*th*, 1883, with various ills. The constipation for which I had treated her had been cured by *Nux* 30 and *Sulphur* 30, but the *fluor albus* was no better. "But then," said she, "there is the neuralgia in my eyes, which I have had for nine years, nothing has ever touched that." The neuralgia complained of was worse in the morning and at the menstrual period.

Thuja 30 (4 in 24). One at night.

I saw her no more till the 8*th* of December, 1883, when she called complaining of too frequent and too profuse menstruation.

"What about the neuralgia?"

"Oh! that is cured; I have not had it since those powders."

Was this a case of vaccinosis?

Patient had been twice vaccinated, and the second time was when she was 15 years old, when it did *not take*. I do not feel so sure that this was a case of vaccinosis, because patient was revaccinated unsuccessfully *after* this neuralgia began, and besides, her mother died of epithelioma, so it may have been merely a case of *sycosis Hahnemanni*. The only certain thing about it is that the neuralgia had lasted nine years, and disappeared after the giving of the *Thuja*.

I have treated a certain number of other cases, with varied disease symptoms, on the hypothesis that I was dealing with vaccinosis, and often with results little short of startling, but I hardly think it would serve any useful purpose to multiply examples. The foregoing observations embody and exemplify all that is essential of what I have observed and thought on the subject; if other physicians will follow on the same lines the reward will be theirs and mine; and if they will not, then the reward still is mine in this that I have cured very obstinate cases of disease by reckoning with vaccinosis as a clinical fact, and as a man I could not do less than lay what I believe I know on the subject before the world. It remains for others to judge whether the work was worth doing.

Although I had fully intended citing no more cases of vaccinosis and its cure by *Thuja*, still the following very recent observation is really too telling to be left out.

Observation xx.

On January 25*th*, 1884, I was requested to see a lady in a well-known London Square. She is a trifle over fifty, healthy looking, and enjoying good health except for her *headaches*. These headaches were the bane of her life, as any extra exertion, worry, or work put her out and brought them on or exacerbated them. A few visitors at her house, her ordinary social duties, a dinner, an evening at the theatre, a little meeting for benevolent purposes, an uncivil servant—each and all put her *hors de combat* with her headache. She had had them "every few days and ever since she could remember, but greatly increased in severity during the past three years." She did not expect to be cured; "at my age, and after so many years," said this lady.

Moreover, she did *not* believe in homœopathy, "no, not in the least, but I have tried all the best doctors and they have failed, and hearing from Lady ———, that you were specially good at headaches, I determined to send for you."

"Vaccinated?" "Oh! yes, five or six times; has not taken for years; do you think I had better be done again?"

Thuja Occidentalis 30.

On Feb. 9*th* I called.—"Oh, I am better, I have only had one headache—two days after I began with your powders—and I am very much less nervous." To continue the medicine.

March 2*nd*.—"I have not had any headache at all, although I have been doing just the very things that always bring them on; I have the greatest confidence in homœopathy, &c."

These are, professional brother, what I conceive to be clinical facts. The lady had had headaches for more than 30 years; I gave her *Thuja*, and the headaches departed, and thus far have not returned.

But what are facts to me may be faddles to you, all laws of evidence to the contrary notwithstanding.

SOME REMARKS ON HOMŒOPROPHYLAXIS.

In the April number, 1884, of the *Homœopathic World*, there appeared the following communication to the Editor:—

DR. SKINNER ON M. PASTEUR'S HOMŒOPATHY.

DEAR SIR,—If the italicised is not Homœopathy, what is it?

THOS. SKINNER, M.D.

25, Somerset St., W., Feb. 27, 1884.

M. PASTEUR'S EXPERIMENTS.

M. Pasteur made an interesting communication to the Paris Academy of Sciences on Monday in relation to canine madness. His experiments had shown him that an injection in the region of the skull of the virus of rabies always produced the malady in an acute form, but that an injection in the veins only occasionally had acute results, being often followed by chronic affection only, without barking or ferocity. If a dog were inoculated with fragments of marrow or of nerve taken from a mad dog, the disease would be communicated. *M. Pasteur further stated that he had rendered twenty dogs proof against the disease by inoculating them with other virus than the virus of rabies.* Fowls and pigeons injected with the latter became affected, but soon recovered spontaneously.

"If the italicised is not Homœopathy, what is it?" Just so, *what* is it?

I think a little reflection will shew that it belongs in the sphere of preventive medicine, and is not homœopathy, *i.e.*, it is an extension of the principle of similars to the prevention of disease.

Many other ardent homœopaths besides Dr. Skinner have claimed that vaccination is a proof of the truth of homœopathy; that it is, in fact, part and parcel of it. Evidently this is from the want of a little thought on the subject, since it must be manifest that such is quite impossible, for the simple reason that homœopathy is a system of *curing*—*similia similibus curantur*—whereas vaccination is not a *curative* measure at all, but a *preventive one*. And since prevention is, admittedly, *better* than cure, it must follow that it cannot be the *same*; therefore, vaccination is not homœopathy, though I shall suggest that it might fitly be termed *Homœoprophylaxis*, inasmuch as vaccinia and variola are similar pustular diseases, and the former being preventive of the latter, it may be in obedience to the principle—LIKE PREVENTS LIKE. Being a question of prophylaxis, it cannot be classed in *any* system of *cure*. And that likes *are* prevented by likes, *I* could adduce very many examples to shew, did the narrow limits of this little treatise admit of it. Here it must suffice to differentiate between homœopathy and homœoprophylaxis, and to endeavour in a very general way to study a little the true nature of the latter as exemplified in vaccination and analogous facts such as Pasteur's inoculations.

Giving a variolous patient vaccine pus, or lymph (vaccininum), wherewith *to cure* his small-pox, that is homœopathy, and we have ample testimony that it will thus act if given in refracted dose, and thus acting, it can hardly be other than homœopathic in such action. The law of similars is the groundwork of both; in the one case to prevent, and in the other to cure.

M. Pasteur and others, by their inoculations, are empirically labouring to extend homœoprophylaxis in the line initiated by Jennerian vaccination, or rather it is a revival of the old inoculation for small-pox, and on a line with syphilization.

We are here met by the dose-question, just the same as we are in homœopathy, or the treatment of disease by the light of the law of likes. By the clear light of this same law will *preventive* medicine also have to march.

But the dose?

Jennerian vaccination is in accordance with the principle of homœoprophylaxis, though only enunciated as an empiric fact by Jenner, and ever since practised as such. Pasteur gets, perhaps, a little further by advancing along the line of "cultivating." One cannot help wondering, however, how much Pasteur knows of isopathy and of homœopathy. We will return to M. Pasteur's experiments presently.

Nature of Homœoprophylaxis.

The *prevention* of disease according to the law of similars—homœoprophylaxis—is still struggling with its swaddling clothes, but we may reflect on the following:—

Two similar diseases will affect the organism similarly: they will affect the same parts, organs, or tissues, and in a like manner.

If we call the two diseases *a* and *b*, and the organism O, then if *a* fall upon O, and affect it positively (positive effect = *c*), this effect of *a* upon O, *c*, will be like the effect of *b* (= *d*), for *a* and *b* are alike.

Now if we admit that the similarity between *a* and *b* is enough to render them effectively equal, potentially congruent, then we should say $a = b$, and therefore $c = d$. Consequently $O + a = O + b$, and $O + c = O + d$.

That is the question for the solution of which we must appeal to scientific experiment, both at the bedside and in the laboratory, as well as to abstract reasoning.

It has frequently appeared to the writer that *time* and *quantity* (dose), are not duly reckoned with in the question of the efficacy or inefficacy of Jennerian vaccination; and Pasteur seems also to lose sight of both factors in his own experiments. The great mass of medical men firmly believe that vaccination protects against variola; and, that vaccinia and variola *are* ALIKE is quite certain; it is only the *degree* of the likeness that can be subject of dispute, for both are pyrexial pustular diseases.

Statistics of a number of years, nevertheless, shew that variola is, in the aggregate, about as deadly as ever, allowing for a natural decrease in its vis by age; this cannot be controverted, so much must be conceded to the anti-vaccinators.

And yet, given groups of individuals are evidently protected *for the time* from variola by vaccination, and the more recent the vaccinia the greater the temporary protection, *provided the effect of the vaccination be not too great, in which case there will be a homœoprophylactic aggravation, and then there will not only be no protective power, but on the contrary the vaccinate will be predisposed to it*, *i.e.*, instead of a positive and a negative eliminating one another we shall have two positives to be added together.

Let us express the difference between a vaccinated and an unvaccinated individual by the algebraic quantity *x*. Now, what is the nature of *x?* Is it positive or negative? *Quoad* perfect health it is negative, but *quoad* the organismic individual it is positive, if a diseased condition can be said to be a positive one.

To begin with, it is inconceivable that *x* should be a CONSTANT FACTOR, which is evidently the general assumption; it must be an always lessening quantity, and *x* might thus be initially congruent with variola, while it may at any subsequent point be incongruent. This really expresses the sum of human experience on the question of the efficacy or inefficacy of Jennerian vaccination, though it is not apprehended; whence the cry for re-vaccination *coup sur coup* on the one hand, and the want of faith in vaccination on the other, both positions being readily comprehensible if the effect of vaccination be recognised as an *inconstant* factor.

And from these considerations it must be manifest that the protection afforded by vaccination will be different in different individuals, and diminishingly different in the same individual, and always growing less and less until it is *nil*. Thus *x* might to-day be preventively equal to variola in an endemic form, but not equal to it in epidemic form. In other words the protection afforded by *x* is relative and contingent. Moreover, if the vaccinosis be too great, *i.e.*, too powerfully diseasing, it not only cannot protect, but must actually add fuel to the flames.

We thus appear to arrive at the conclusion that vaccination does relatively and contingently protect from small-pox as a disease, but nevertheless, the mortality from small-pox remains in the aggregate the same, but in a greater percentage. That is to say, fewer people probably get small-pox, but the absolute number of deaths is not affected, or is greater.

In pro-vaccinational and anti-vaccinational literature, *morbility* and *mortality* are commonly confounded together. We have no means of knowing how many people *get* small-pox, either absolutely or proportionately, we only know how many *die* of it. Therefore *all* the vaccination statistics are wide of the mark except perhaps those in certain hospitals. The pro-vaccinators maintain that vaccination protects from variola because they see that, as a general rule, the vaccinated do not get small-pox. The anti-vaccinists say, "Oh! but a good many of your vaccinated persons *do* get small-pox nevertheless, and the mortality from small-pox is as great as ever, or greater than ever!" Both sides are honest; both are apparently dealing with facts; both are striving after truth, and collectively they expend enough human energy to enrich a nation or colonize a continent. Where then is the missing link?

While writing this, an ardent bacterist, Dr. H. Thomas, of Llandudno, very kindly sends me a clipping from the *Athenæum* of March 15*th*, 1884. It run thus:

> M. PASTEUR and his fellow labourers communicated to the Académie des Sciences on the 25*th* of February the important fact that by inoculation with virus taken from mad dogs they can render all dogs absolutely safe from the effects of rabies, in whatever way and in whatever quantity the virus may be administered.

This is the same fact referred to by Dr. Skinner further back.

But we find no principle enunciated here by the *Athenæum;* nevertheless, the results must be in obedience to the *law of similars in prophylactics*—homœoprophylaxis.

Here M. Pasteur and his fellow-workers, just the same as the Jennerian vaccinators, and the anti-vaccinators—here, I say, they practically ignore the element *time*, and the altering nature of the protection. When people speak of "the necessity of *re*-vaccination, because vaccination loses its effect," *time* is roughly reckoned with, but an arbitrary limit is set entirely devoid of any scientific basis.

On the other hand it has been often noticed that a healthy person gets variola soon after vaccination, which to my mind militates in no wise against a belief in the protective power of vaccination, but is to be interpreted as meaning that the vaccinial infection was more than enough; just the same as a *little Aconite* will *lessen* feverishness, while *much Aconite* will make the feverishness worse.

Continuing now to let x stand for the difference between a vaccinate and a non-vaccinate, we must keep well before our minds that x represents the remaining effects of a disease—vaccinosis—and this is *not* a constant quantity; in an otherwise healthy person it must be continually growing less and less, and finally become extinct. Therefore, in order to determine whether vaccination protects against variola or not, we must first have the date of the vaccination in each case of varioloid or small-pox in the vaccinate. Were a considerable number of such cases tabulated we might arrive at some idea as to how long a given vaccination continues to affect the individual sufficiently for the vaccinosis to leave no room for variola, provided always that the vaccinations were unipotential.

Is it possible for Vaccination to be contingently Effective, and yet for the Mortality from Small-pox to be Greater?

This question crops up and presents itself to one's mind thus:

Vaccination protects from variola say the vaccinators.

Quoth the anti-vaccinators—That is impossible, because some of those who have been vaccinated *do* get variola, and the mortality from variola has actually increased, so where is the prevention?

How can these things be?

Let us ponder these points. And first of all let us not confound morbility with mortality. We really want three words to express our meaning well. Firstly, mortality, or the number of deaths; secondly, *morbidity*, or the quantity of ill-health of the living; and thirdly, *morbility*, or the number of those who actually take a given disease. I ask forgiveness for this word-coining; no one need use the words if they are needless or objectionable, but it seems to me that these three ideas must be accurately expressed if we are to adequately discuss the question.

In judging of the ill-effects of vaccination, only the mortality is considered as a general rule by the pro-vaccinists. By giving attention to vaccinational morbidity (the vaccinosis of this little treatise), I have been enabled to do some notably good clinical work, and I put the facts observed before the world as a duty, and really unwillingly, as I am sure to be much misunderstood, but that cannot be helped, and besides I am now wandering away from my text.

Before we can scientifically

reckon with vaccination we must take accurate account of the morbility as well as of the mortality and morbidity. The practical physician alone has the necessary scope for making observations in respect of the morbidity arising from vaccination, *i.e.*, vaccinosis. Unfortunately it is completely ignored as a general rule.

Any statistician can observe and arrange the facts relating to its morbility, and the Registrar General might be got to deal with them as he does with those relating to mortality. But, I must submit that mortality statistics alone without morbility statistics cannot possibly lead to any real settlement of the vaccination question, for we want to know not only how many die of small-pox, but also how many *get* it and get over it.

Herein, it seems to me, lies the kernel of the nut.

And not only do we want to know how many get small-pox and recover, and how many get it and die of it, but also what is the morbidity of those protected by the vaccination.

What is the ordinary liability of the perfectly healthy to catch small-pox, *i.e.*, what is their prospective morbility, morbidity, and mortality?

Assuming that vaccination does protect, relatively and contingently, what do we pay for the protection, not in money, but in vaccinial morbidity, or vaccinosis?

It seems to me probable that

ordinary Jennerian vaccination is not efficiently protective in those whose proneness to catch small-pox is very great, while it *is* efficiently protective where the proneness to catch small-pox is less.

If we reflect upon this for a while we shall see that there is nothing unreasonable in this proposition.

The un-vaccinated are not equally prone to catch small-pox; we vaccinate them all *alike*.

Now is it even conceivable that the vaccination has rendered them *equally* immune, when some of the *un*-vaccinated were *already* immune?

My line of argument here stands thus:—Vaccination is preventive of small-pox when the proneness to catch it is small; and when the proneness to catch it is small, those who do get small pox do *not* die of it, therefore vaccination affects the *morbility* rather that the mortality of small-pox. I refer to ordinary Jennerian vaccination, and not to microposic homœoprophylaxis.

If I am right then we can affirm on aprioristic grounds that ordinary macroposic vaccination will diminish morbility but *increase* the mortality, *i.e.*, fewer will get it, but more will die: the mortality will be greater.

How so?

Vaccination is a homœoprophylactic diseasing measure: one disease is given to prevent a like one,—vaccinia to prevent variola. If the diseasing process of vaccination fail to protect, then the vaccinated person will be *more* likely to die because there is the homœoprophylactic *aggravation:* the two diseases combine to kill the patient just the same as too much of the homœopathic remedy will aggravate the disease to which it is highly homœopathic; with, perhaps, the like result.

This is manifest, for in vaccinating a person we are *diseasing* him; we communicate vaccinosis to him: if he, in addition to the vaccinosis, now get small-pox, he is the more likely to die the worse he has the vaccinosis.

If *y* represent the prospective mortality of the unvaccinated, and

x the difference between the vaccinated and the unvaccinated, *i.e.*, vaccinosis, then the chances of dying of the vaccinated person who gets small-pox are $y + x$.

Against the hypothesis that vaccination may be protective in some cases (relatively and contingently), and add fuel to the flames in others, *i.e.*, decrease the morbility and increase the mortality. Against this hypothesis it will be objected that the mortality is much greater in variola than it is in varioloid. This, I submit, proves nothing, because the unvaccinated belong almost exclusively to the social residuum in whom all diseases are relatively very fatal. Vaccination has been *comme il faut* now for many years, and hence almost everybody who is anybody has been vaccinated. Nearly all the anti-vaccinists have themselves been vaccinated. Now that the mental *élite* of the world are rising against vaccination, I venture to foretell that in the future the mortality in *their* unvaccinated offspring will be very small; probably only those who inherit the PURULENT DIATHESIS will die, and many of these would be saved if homœopathically handled, or homœoprophylactically vaccinated in refracted dose.

DYNAMIC OR MICROPOSIC HOMŒOPROPHYLAXIS.

When I began with this little essay I meant it to be on the one hand a contribution to the clinical history of *Thuja Occidentalis*, and on the other a plea for the recognition of the clinical importance of vaccinosis, particularly in chronic neurotic headaches. But as I went on I felt impelled to say a few words on the subject of what I have called homœoprophylaxis, and now I cannot bring myself to conclude without dipping a little into the dynamics of preventive medicine according to the law of likes.

Strewn about in literature there are examples of small-dose homœoprophylaxis; see Hahnemann's little essay on Belladonna, for example, at the very birth of Hahnemannian homœopathy.

Then vaccine "lymph"—pus—

has been dynamized *more homœopathico* and given as a prophylactic against small-pox in epidemic times, and apparently with effect. *Thuja Occidentalis* has been used in like manner by more than one homœopathic practitioner, and they claim that it is effective. The eminent Dr. David Wilson, of London, has, I hear, long used *Thuja*, in dynamic dose, as a sure preventive of variola.

Speaking for myself, I have for the last nine years been in the habit of using vaccine matter, in the thirtieth homœopathic centesimal potency, whenever small-pox was about, and I have thus far not seen anyone so treated get variola.

Dr. Massoto inoculated the diphtheritic exudation in an epidemic of diphtheria, and that with success.

It seems to me that the requirement of the age is to *systematize* the prevention of disease according to the law of similars, AND IN DYNAMIC DOSE. Clearly the dynamic dose is ESSENTIAL, or at any rate the very small dose, for otherwise the homœoprophylactic aggravation would be a serious detriment in every way. It is easy to see that M. Pasteur and his fellow workers are sailing down straight on this rock, whereon they are sure to suffer shipwreck.

M. Pasteur's latest communications to the Académie des Sciences are in substance as follows:—

"If the virus of rabies be transmitted from the dog to the monkey, and then from monkey to monkey, it will be found that after each transmission the virulence of the virus has become enfeebled. If the virus thus enfeebled be re-transmitted to a dog, or an animal of that species, it will remain still attenuated. By a few transmissions of the virus from monkey to monkey, there can easily be obtained a virus so attenuated as shall never communicate, by hypodermic inoculations, the disease to a dog. Inoculations by trepanning of such virus will likewise produce no result; but an animal will, notwithstanding, be rendered thereby proof against the disease. The virulence of the virus becomes, on the contrary, augmented in its passage from rabbit to rabbit. If a dog be inoculated with virus thus augmented in power, a far more intense form of the disease will be manifested than that apparent in ordinary canine madness, and it will invariably prove fatal."

By applying these and other observations, M. Pasteur obtained virus of different degrees of virulence, and succeeded, by inoculations of the milder qualities, in preserving animals from the effects of more active and mortal kinds. For example, after several days longer than the shortest incubation term, M. Pasteur extracted virus from the head of a rabbit which had died of the disease, and inoculated successively two other rabbits. Each time a dog was inoculated with the virus, which, as has been seen, would increase each time in virulence. The result was that the dog was ultimately rendered capable of bearing a virus of mortal strength, and became absolutely proof against canine virus. M. Pasteur anticipates that the time is still distant when canine madness will be extinguished by vaccination, but pending that consummation, he feels pretty certain that he will be able to avert the consequences of a bite from a mad dog. He says:—"Thanks to the duration of incubation after a bite, I have every reason to believe that patients can be rendered insusceptible before the mortal malady has had time to declare itself." M. Pasteur stated, in conclusion, that he had solicited the Minister of Education to appoint a Commission to test his experiments. He added:—

"The principal experiment that I shall attempt will consist in taking from my kennels twenty dogs insusceptible to the disease, and placing the same in comparison with twenty ordinary dogs I shall then have all these forty dogs bitten by a number of dogs in a rabid state. If the facts that I have enunciated are exact, the twenty dogs that I believe to be proof against the disease will remain healthy, while the other twenty will become affected. For a second experiment no less decisive, I propose to place before the Commission twenty vaccinated and twenty un-vaccinated dogs. All the forty I shall then inoculate in the most sensitive parts with virus taken from a rabid dog. The twenty vaccinated dogs will resist, and the other twenty will all die of madness, either paralytic or furious."

This is as far as M. Pasteur has got at present, and his labours clearly tend in the direction of homœoprophylaxis and homœopathy; but time and dose are not duly reckoned with. The fatal fallacy underlying the whole thing is regarding the immunity produced by Jennerian or Pasteurian vaccination *as a constant factor*, whereas it is a constantly diminishing one, and must in the nature of things be so.

As a last word I would put in a plea for homœoprophylactic vaccination, or what might be termed homœopathic vaccination. That is to say, the vaccine matter is to be prepared as a homœopathic remedy, and to be given by the mouth, in dynamic dose as the homœoprophylactic. Pasteur's attenuating it by poisoning a series of animals is ridiculous; an ordinary vial will do just as well. It is with virus thus attenuated that I used to treat myself when I was attending small-pox instead of being re-vaccinated. I used to treat my family and others with whom I was compelled to associate in the same way. None of us ever took small-pox.

In magnis voluisse sat est.